Medical Mnemonics for the Family Nurse Practitioner

Nachole Johnson

Illustrated by Murhiel Caberte

Copyright 2016 Nachole Johnson and ReNursing Publishing Company.

ALL RIGHTS RESERVED.

Disclaimer

Although the author and publisher have made every effort to ensure the information provided in this book were correct at press time, the author and publisher do not assume and hereby disclaim any liability to any party for any loss, damage, or disruption caused by errors or omissions, whether such errors or omissions result from negligence, accident, or any other cause.

This book is not intended as the substitute for the legal advice or consultation of attorneys. The reader should regularly consult an attorney in matters relating to his/her business that may require legal advisement.

All rights are reserved. No part of this publication may be reproduced, distributed, more transmitted in any form or by any means, including photocopying, recording, or other electronic or means, including photocopying, recording, or any other electronic or mechanical methods, without the prior written permission of the publisher, except in no commercial use permitted uses permitted by copyright law.

ISBN: 9781542711005

Printed in the United States of America

10 9 8 7 6 5 4 3 2 1

Table of Contents

Why I Wrote This Book ....
Chapter 1 Common Abbreviations 1
Chapter 2 Documentation Basics 7
Chapter 3: Dermatology 15
Chapter 4: Neurology 21
Chapter 5: EENT 25
Chapter 6: Cardiovascular 29
Chapter 7: Pulmonary 35
Chapter 8: Gastrointestinal 39
Chapter 9: Genitourinary 43
Chapter 10: Endocrine 45
Chapter 11: Hematology 49
Chapter 12: Immunology 53
Chapter 13: Musculoskeletal 57
Chapter 14: Reproductive 61
Chapter 15: Pediatrics 65
Chapter 16: Psychosocial 71
Chapter 17: Pharmacology 75
Chapter 18: Top 25 Drugs in Family Practice 79

Why I Wrote This Book

There's a lot to learn while you are in nurse practitioner school. Because of the time pressure, I really appreciated anything that would help me get through school. I've always been a visual learner, and it is easy for me to pick up information if I draw out pictures or play with words to make learning a complex issue easier. I loved using mnemonics when I was in nursing school, and that continued when I went to graduate school for my Family Nurse Practitioner degree.

I found it was easy for me to remember silly sayings during the test that would remind me of the right answer. Turns out, many other people like mnemonics too! I decided to write a book specifically for the Nurse Practitioner field. It is a bit of a cross between what you would expect from a book for nurses and one geared toward physicians.

Use this book as a guide to memorize common concepts and as a refresher for ones you haven't used in a while. Even when you are out of school and in practice, it is sometimes difficult to remember a concept you haven't used since the final exam. This is normal and happens to nurse practitioners and physicians alike. I still use silly mnemonics to remember things like the cranial nerves "**O**n **O**ld **O**lympus **T**owering **T**ops **A** **F**in **A**nd **G**erman **V**iewed **S**ome **H**ops," anyone?

Use this book while you are in school and as a refresher when you finish. I've included extras for Nurse Practitioners like medical abbreviations, documentation basics, and a list of commonly prescribed medications in family practice. Have fun, learn, and enjoy!

- *Nachole*

Chapter 1
Common Abbreviations

ABG	Arterial Blood Gas
a.c.	Before meals
add	adduction
ADL	Activities of Daily Living
A. Fib.	Atrial fibrillation
AKA	Above the knee amputation
AMA	Against medical advice
A&O	Alert and oriented
A/P	Anterior-posterior
b.i.d.	Twice a day
BKA	Below the knee amputation
bm	Bowel movement
BM	Bone marrow
BP	Blood pressure
bs	Bowel sounds
BS	Breath sounds
bx	Biopsy
CA, ca	Cancer
CABG	Coronary artery bypass graft
cal	calorie
CC	Chief complaint
CHI	Closed Head injury
CN	Cranial Nerve
CNS	Central nervous system
c/o	Complaints of
CPAP	Continuous positive airway pressure
CPR	Cardiopulmonary resuscitation
CSF	Cerebral spinal fluid
CT	Computerized tomography

CXR	Chest x-ray
d	day
d/c	discontinue
DNR	Do not resuscitate
DOB	Date of birth
DOE	Dyspnea on exertion
d/t	Due to
Dx	Diagnosis
ECG	Electrocardiogram
EKG	Electrocardiogram
EEG	Electroencephalogram
EMG	electromyogram
ENT	Ear, nose, throat
ext	external, exterior
FH	Family history
fl, fld	Fluid
f/u	Follow-up
Fx	Fracture
gest.	Gestation
glu	Glucose
GTT	Glucose tolerance test
GYN	Gynecology
h	Hour
H/A	Headache
Hb.	Hemoglobin
h.s.	bedtime
h/o	History of
Hx	History
ICP	Intercranial pressure
incr.	Increased
int.	Internal
I&O	Intake and Output
lac.	Laceration
liq	Liquid
LBW	Low Birth Weight
L.O.C.	Loss of consciousness, Level of consciousness, Laxative of choice
LOS	Length of Stay

LP	Lumbar Puncture
LUE	Left upper extremity
m,M	married, male, mother, murmur, meter, mass, molar
max.	Maximum
mets.	Metastasis
min	Minute
MRI	Magnetic resonance Imaging
MRSA	Methicillin-resistant Staphylococcus Aureus
MVA	Motor Vehicle Accident
n.	Nerve
NAD	No abnormality detected, no apparent distress
neur.	Neurology
NG	Nasogastric
NKDA	No known drug allergies
NPO	Nothing by mouth
NST	Non-stress test
N&V	Nausea and vomiting
NVD	Nausea, vomiting, diarrhea
o	none, without, oral
OB/OBG	Obstetrics
Obs	Observation
OH	Occupational history
oint.	Ointment
O.M.	Otitis Media
O.M.E.	Otitis Media with effusion
OTC	Over-the-counter
p&a	Percussion and auscultation
palp.	Palpate, palpated, palpable
Path	Pathology
PA	Posterior - Anterior view on x-ray
p/c, p.c.	after meals
PE	Physical Exam
	Pulmonary embolism
PH	Past History
PET	Positron Emission Tomography
PHYS.	Physical, Physiology
PI	Present Illness, Pulmonary insufficiency
PN	Poorly Nourished

Pneu.	Pneumo, pneumonia
p.o.	By mouth
p.o.d.	postoperative day
prod.	Productive
Prog.	Prognosis
prosth.	Prosthesis
PSH	Past surgical history
pt., Pt.	Patient
PT	Physical therapy
PWB	Partial weight bearing
q	every
q.h.	every hour
q.i.d.	four times daily
qt.	Quart
R, r	Right
RA	rheumatoid arthritis, right atrium
rad.	Radial
RAtx	Radiation therapy
RCA	Right coronary artery
RDS	Respiratory distress syndrome
RLE	Right lower extremely
ROM	Range of motion, Rupture of membranes, Right Otitis Media
ROS	Review of systems
Rt.	right
RT	Radiation therapy Respiratory therapy
RUE	Right Upper extremity
s	Without
s.c.	Subcutaneously
Sx	Symptoms
sys.	system
T	temperature
T&A	Tonsils and adenoids tonsillectomy and adeniodectomy
tab.	tablet
TAH	Total abdominal hysterectomy

TB	Tuberculosis
TBI	Traumatic brain injury
tbsp.	tablespoon
temp	Temperature
tsp.	teaspoon
Tx	Treatment
U/A	urinalysis
Ur.	Urine
u/s.	Ultrasound
UTI	Urinary tract infection
V	vein
VA	visual acuity
vag	vagina
vit.	Vitamin
VS	Vital signs

Chapter 2
Documentation Basics

Proper documenting and through documenting are a necessary evil of your daily job as an NP. It can be hard to remember everything when it comes to interacting with your patients on a daily basis
especially when you are just starting out. Documentation mnemonics can help you with your daily charting
for both keeping facts straight for medical records and any potential legal issues that could arise.

Basic NP Note Format

Subjective: What the patient says

Objective: What you observe

Assessment: What you think is going on

Plan: What you intend to do about it

Abdominal Assessment

DR. GERM

- **D**istention (liver problems, bowel obstruction)
- **R**idgidity (bleeding)
- **G**uarding: Muscular tension when touched
- **E**visceration/Ecchymosis
- **R**ebound tenderness (infection)
- **M**asses

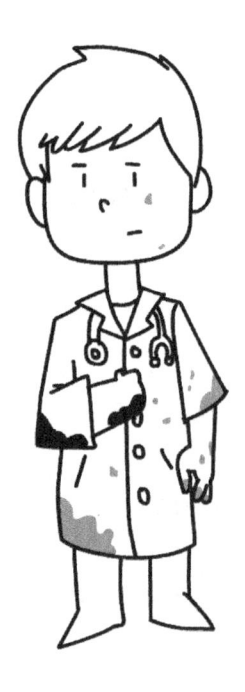

Abdomen exam: I Assess Peoples Paunches
- **I**nspection
- **A**uscultation
- **P**alpate
- **P**ercussion

Pain assessment

Site

Onset

Character

Radiation

Associations

Time

Exacerbating/relieving factors

Severity

"Wisdom begins in wonder."- Socrates

Mental state examination: Elements in order - **"Assessed Mental State To Be Positively Clinically Unremarkable."**
- **A**ppearance and behavior [observed state clothing, grooming]
- **M**ood [recent spirit]
- **S**peech [rate form content]
- **T**hinking [thoughts perceptions]
- **B**ehavioral abnormalities
- **P**erception abnormalities
- **C**ognition [time, place, age]
- **U**nderstanding of condition [ideas, expectations, concerns]

Family History: Elements in order - **BALD CHASM**:
- **B**lood pressure (high)
- **A**rthritis
- **L**ung disease
- **D**iabetes
- **C**ancer
- **H**eart Disease
- **A**lcoholism
- **S**troke
- **M**ental health disorders (depression)

Breast history checklist: Elements in order LMNOP
- **L**ump
- **M**ammary changes
- **N**ipple changes
- **O**ther symptoms
- **P**atient risk factors

Medications/allergies
Mnemonic: PILLS

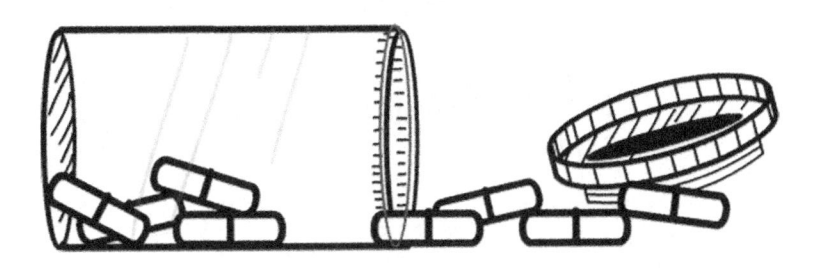

- **P**atient taking meds?
- **I**njections/Insulin/Inhalers (as some patients forget to mention when asked about their medications)
- **ILL**icit drug use
- **S**ensitivities to anything, i.e. allergies

Four point physical assessment of a disease: "I'm A People Person."
- **I**nspection
- **A**uscultation
- **P**ercussion
- **P**alpation

Patient profile: LADDERS

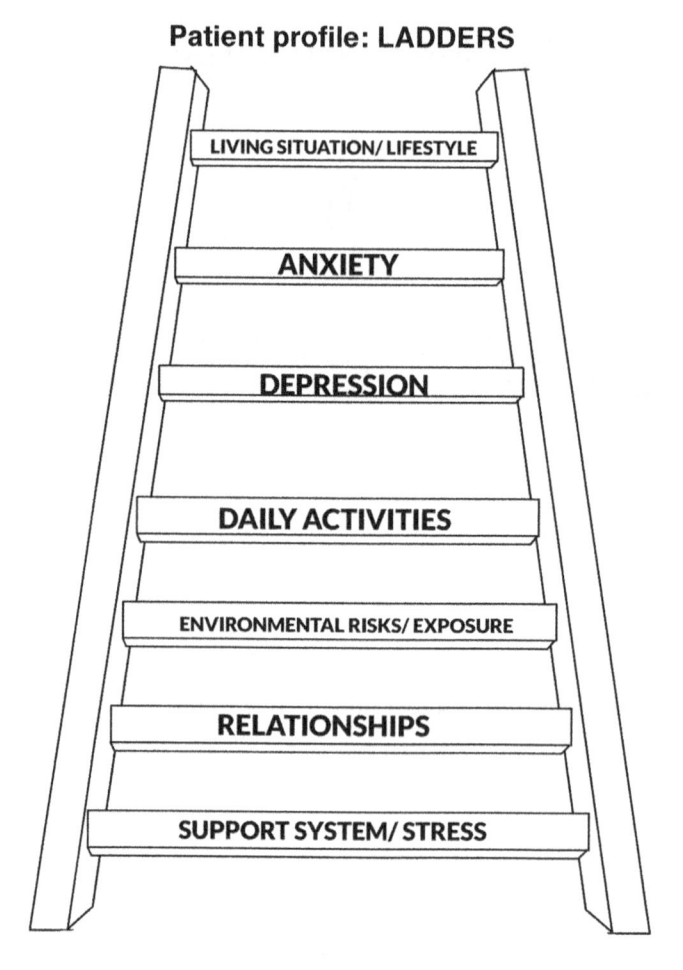

- LIVING SITUATION/ LIFESTYLE
- ANXIETY
- DEPRESSION
- DAILY ACTIVITIES
- ENVIRONMENTAL RISKS/ EXPOSURE
- RELATIONSHIPS
- SUPPORT SYSTEM/ STRESS

- **L**iving situation/Lifestyle
- **A**nxiety
- **D**epression
- **D**aily activities (describe a typical day)
- **E**nvironmental risks/Exposure
- **R**elationships
- **S**upport system/stress

Abbreviations Not to Use

This chapter wouldn't be complete if there wasn't a list of abbreviations you shouldn't use when charting. The Joint Commission has an official "Do Not Use" list when you do your charting. Keep these in mind when documenting.

Do Not Use	Potential Problem	Use Instead
U, u (unit)	Mistaken for "0" (zero), the number "4" (four) or "cc"	Write "unit"
IU (international unit)	Mistaken for IV (intraveneous) or the number 10 (ten)	Write "International Unit"
Q.D., QD, q.d. qd (daily) Q.O.D., QOD, q.o.d., qod (every other day)	Mistaken for each other Period over the Q mistaken for "I" and the "O" mistaken for "I"	Write "daily" Write "every other day"
Trailing zero (X.0 mg)* Lack of leading zero (.X mg)	Decimal point is missed	Write X mg Write 0.X mg
MS MSO4 and MgSO4	Can mean morphine sulfate or magnesium sulfate Confused for one another	Write "morphine sulfate" Write "magnesium sulfate"

Official "Do Not Use" List from JCAHO (www.jointcommission.org)

Chapter 3: Dermatology

Mole trouble: ABCDE
- **A**symmetry
- **B**order irregular
- **C**olor irregular
- **D**iameter usually > 0.5 cm
- **E**levation irregular

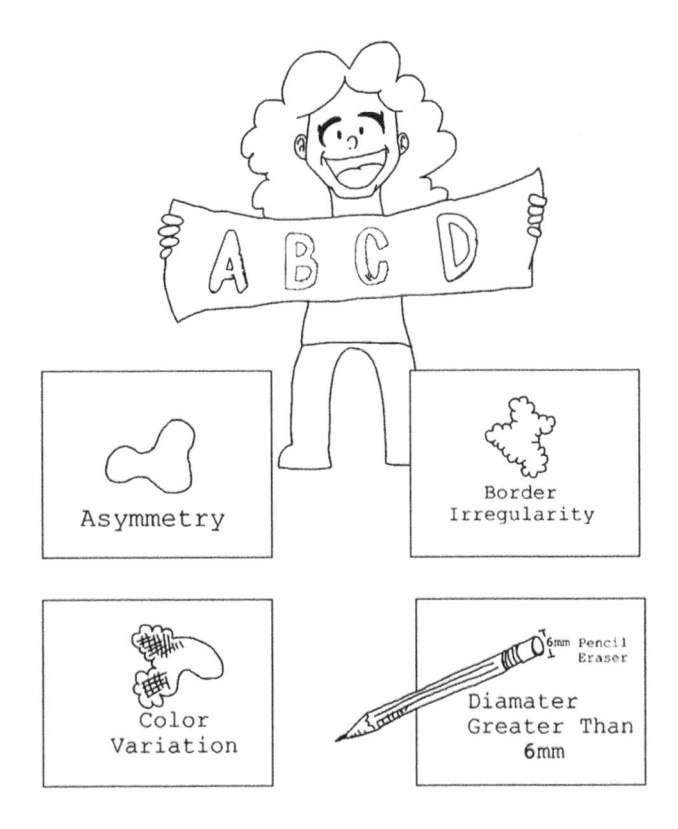

Asymmetry

Border Irregularity

Color Variation

6mm Pencil Eraser

Diamater Greater Than 6mm

Contact dermatitis: CONTACT:
- **C**utaneous type IV reaction
- **O**intments and cosmetics containing lanolin
- **N**ickel
- **T**opical antibiotics (neosporin)
- **A**utosensitization can occur (secondary spread elsewhere)
- **C**hromates (cement, leather)/colophon (plasters, glue, ink)
- **T**opical antihistamines and topical anesthetics (hemorrhoid creams)

Vitiligo: Vitiligo PATCH:
- **P**ityriasis
- **A**lba/ Post-Inflammatory hypo pigmentation, Age-related hypo pigmentation
- **T**inea versicolor/ Tuberous sclerosis (ash leaf macule)
- **C**ongential birthmark
- **H**ansen's (leprosy)

Delayed wound healing: DID NOT HEAL
- **D**rugs
- **I**nfections/Icterus/Ischemia
- **D**iabetes
- **N**utrition
- **O**xygen (hypoxia)
- **T**oxins
- **H**ypothermia/Hyperthermia
- **E**TOH
- **A**cidosis
- **L**ocal anesthetics

Cross reactivity to Latex allergy: BLACK Passion fruit:
- **B**anana
- **L**atex
- **A**vocado
- **C**hestnut
- **K**iwi
- **Pa**ssion fruit

Melanoma Risks – "M RISKS"
- **M**oles that are atypical or dysplastic nevi, Moles that are many in number
- **R**ed hair
- **I**nability to tan
- **S**unburn (especially severe burns before age 14)
- **K**indred (family history)

Oral Ulcer Causes: BUCCAL MUCOSA
- **B**echet's syndrome
- **U**lcers (aphthae)
- **C**andida (Syphills, HIV)
- **C**ontact dermatitis
- **A**brasions and trauma
- **L**ichen planus
- **M**ultiforme (erythema)
- **U**nknown
- **C**hemotherapy
- **O**ral herpes
- **S**quamous cell cancer
- **A**utoimmune diseases (pemphigus, cicatrical phemphoid, discoid lupus)

Diabetes mellitus skin markers: "Xavier Is Giving Nancy Nasty Ipecac."
- Xanthomas
- Infections
- Granuloma annulare
- Necrobiosis lipoidica
- Neuropathic ulcers
- Infection

Skin hyperpigmentation causes: "It's generalized since no part of the skin is SPARED."
- **S**unlight
- **P**regnancy
- **A**ddison's disease
- **R**enal failure
- **E**xcess of iron (hemochromatosis)
- **D**rugs

Pruritus: SCRATCHED
- **S**cabies
- **C**holestasis
- **R**enal
- **A**uto-immune
- **T**umors (Ca)
- **C**razies
- **H**ematology (polycythemia, lymphoma)
- **E**ndocrine (thyroid, parathyroid, iron deficiency)
- **D**rugs, dry skin

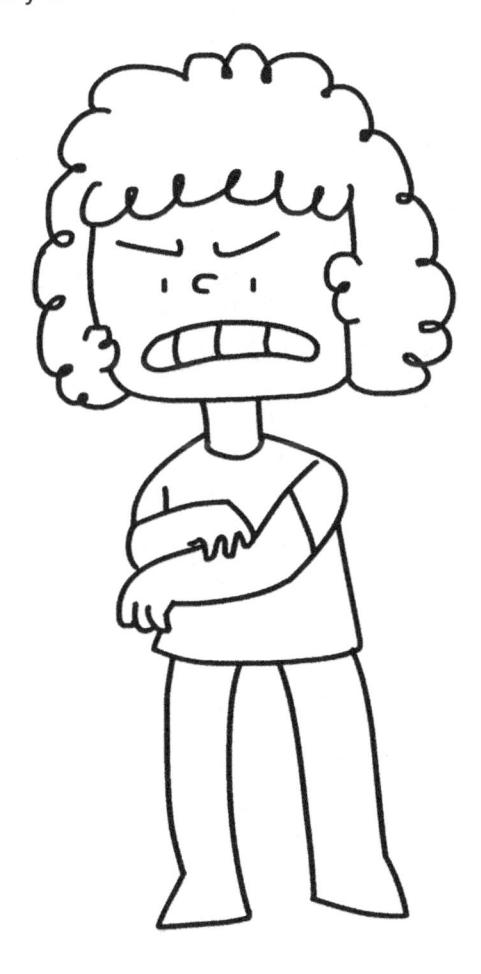

Suture removal times

SUTURE REMOVAL

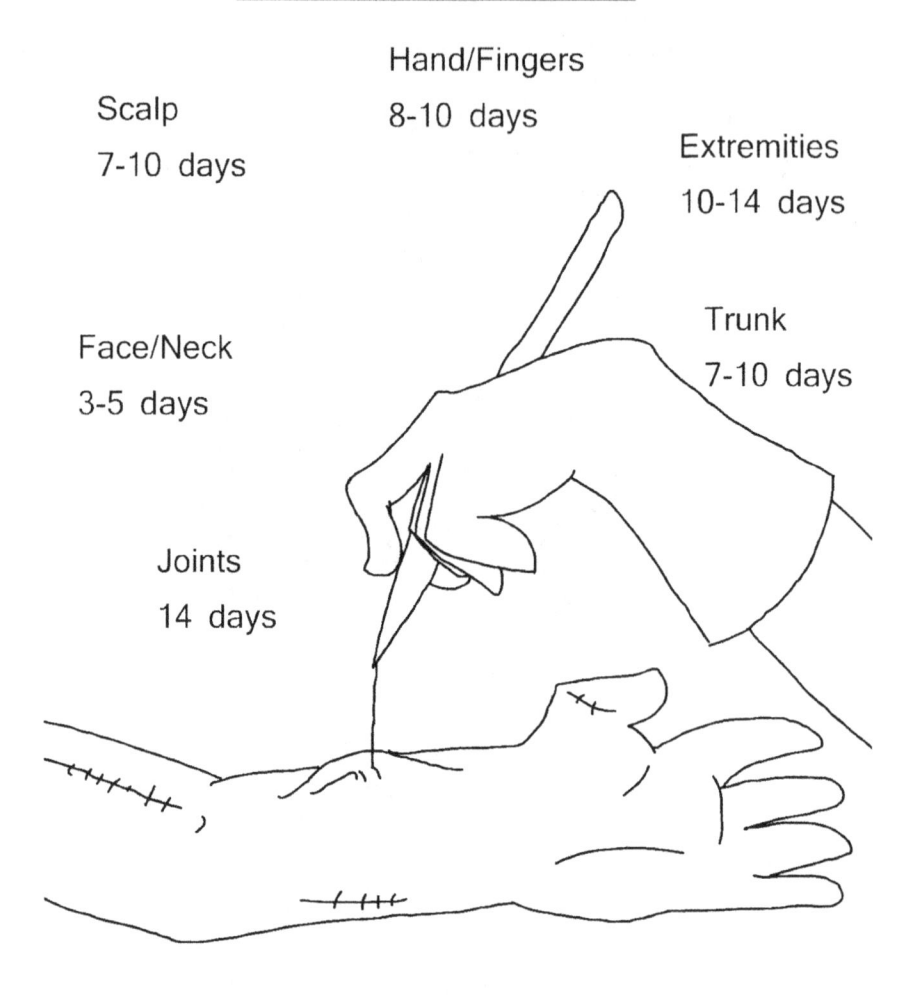

Scalp
7-10 days

Hand/Fingers
8-10 days

Extremities
10-14 days

Face/Neck
3-5 days

Trunk
7-10 days

Joints
14 days

Chapter 4: Neurology

Cranial nerves: "Oh! Oh! Oh! The Times Arrived For All Girls! Vote Against Housework!"

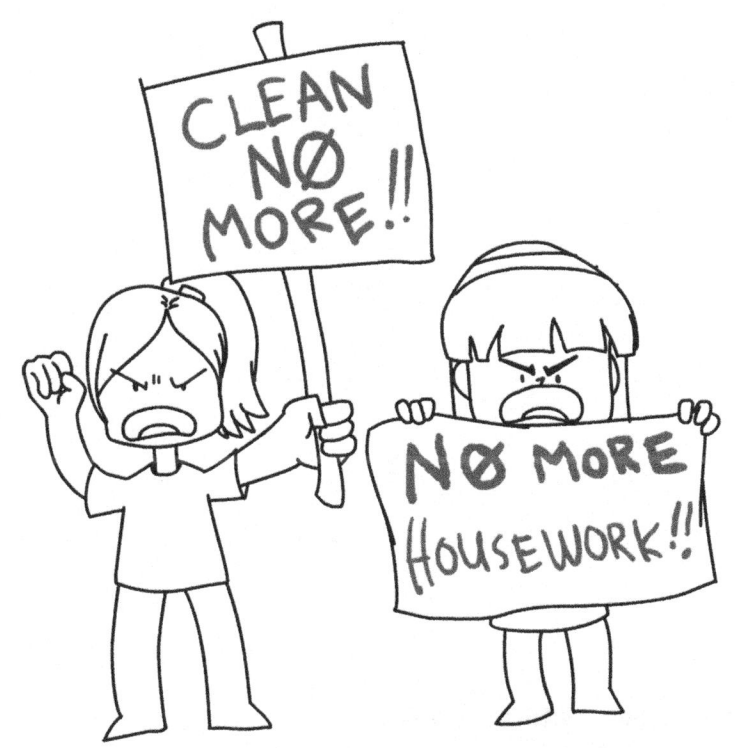

Olfactory
Optic
Oculomotor
Trochlear
Trigeminal
Abducens
Facial

Auditory (vestibulocochlear)
Glossopharyngeal
Vagus
Accessory (spinal)
Hypoglossal

Stroke symptoms: FAST-
- **F**ace
- **A**rms
- **S**peech
- **T**ime

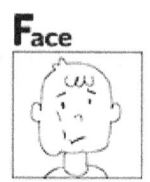

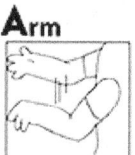

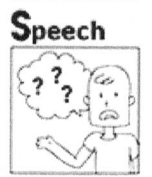

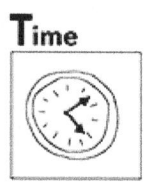

Face

Arm

Speech

Time

Stroke risk factors: HEADS
- **H**ypertension/Hyperlipidemia
- **E**lderly
- **A**trial Fib
- **D**iabetes mellitus/ Drugs (cocaine)
- **S**moking/Sex (male)

Spine (number of vertebrae in each area of spine):
- Breakfast @ 7 (Cervical)
- Lunch @ 12 (Thoracic)
- Dinner @ 5-7 (Lumbar)
- Cocktails @ 3-5 (Coccyx)

Migraine: POUND
- **P**ulsatile
- **O**ne day
- **U**nilateral
- **N**ausea
- Interferes with A**D**L's

Causes of confusion: DEMENTIA
- **D**iabetes/Dementia/Drugs
- **E**pilepsy
- **M**igraine/Multi infarct dementia
- **N**eurologic deficit diseases= BETA
  - **B**leeds
  - **E**ncephalitis
  - **T**umors
  - **A**bscess meningitis
- **T**rauma
- **I**nsulin/Infections
- **A**lzhiemers/Abscess

Parkinson's signs: SMART
- **S**huffling gait
- **M**ask-like face
- **A**kinesia
- **R**igidity
- **T**remor

Causes of Delirium: DELIRIUM
- **D**rugs
- **E**lectrolyte imbalance
- **L**ack of drugs (alcohol withdrawal)
- **I**nfection (UTI, pneumonia)
- **R**educed sensory input (glasses, hearing aides, hospital without clocks or windows)
- **I**ntracranial (stroke)
- **U**rinary or fecal
- **M**I or respiratory

Alzheimer's: 4 A's
- *Amnesia*
- *Agnosia*
- *Apraxia*
- *Aphasia*

Bells Palsy symptoms: BELL'S Palsy:
- **B**link reflex abnormal
- **E**arache
- **L**acrimation [deficient excess]
- **L**oss of taste
- **S**udden onset
- **PALSY** of VII nerve muscles (all symptoms unilateral)

Chapter 5: EENT

Otitis Media causes: Simple Harmonic Melody
- Streptococcus pneumoniae
- Haemophilus Influenza
- Moraxella Catarrhalis

Oralpharyngeal cancers cause: 6 S's:
- Smoking
- Spicy food
- Syphilis
- Spirits
- Sore tooth
- Sepsis

Nasopharyngeal carcinoma causes: NOSE
- Neck mass
- Obstructed nasal passage
- Serous otitis media external
- Epistaxis or drainage

Influenza clinical manifestations: "Having Flu Symptoms Can Make My Children A Nightmare."
- Headache
- Fever
- Sore throat
- Chills
- Myalgias
- Malaise
- Cough
- Anorexia
- Nasal congestion

Strep throat score NO FACE:
- **NO** cough: no cough: no cough is +1
- **F**ever: has fever is +1
- **A**ge: <5 years=-; 15-45 years =0; > 45 years= +1
- **C**ervical nodes: Palpable is +1
- **E**xudate: Tonsillar exudate is +1.

Scoring interpretation:
Score 0-1: No strep throat
Score 1-3: Possible strep throat, do a swab test.
Score 4-5: Strep throat is likely. So treat empirically.

Ear drops: direction to pull ear when instilling
- For an grown **UP** it is **UP**
- For a chil**D** it is **D**own

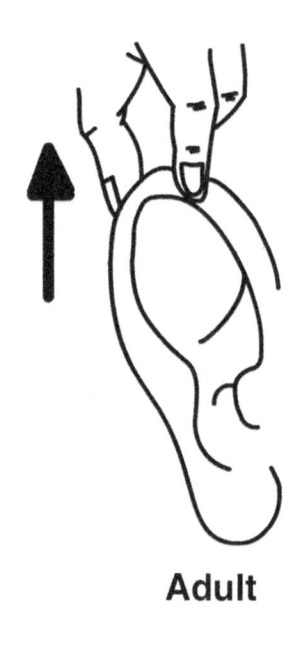

Adult

Child

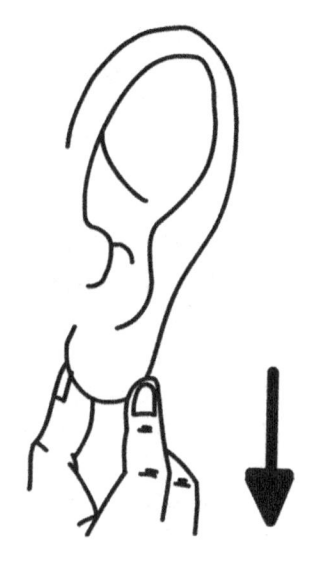

Sinusitis symptoms: "Polly Plays The Harmonic Clarinet Really Nicely"
- Pain
- Postnasal discharge
- Tenderness
- Headache
- Constitutional symptoms
- Redness & edema of cheek
- Nasal discharge

Menieres Disease: DVT
- Deafness
- Vertigo
- Tinnitus

Hemoptysis causes: CAVITATES
- CHF
- Airway disease (bronchiectatsis)
- Vasculitits/Vascular malformations
- Infection (TB)
- Trauma
- Anticoagulation
- Tumor
- Embolism
- Stomach

Clinical features of mumps: SOAP
- Salpingitis
- Orchitis/Oophritis
- Aseptic meningitis
- Pancreatitis

Clinical presentation of conjunctivitis - Mnemonic: BURN
- **B**urning and lacrimation along with itching and possibly photophobia
- **U**sually bilateral- if unilateral consider another differential diagnosis
- **R**ed and inflamed conjunctiva; eyelids may be stuck together with purulent discharge
- **N**ormally self-limiting can be treated with antibiotics

Chapter 6: Cardiovascular

A Fib causes: PIRATES
- **P**ulmonary: PE
- **I**atrogenic COPD
- **R**heumatic heart: mitral regurgitation
- **A**therosclerotic: MI, CAD
- **T**hyroid: hypothyroid
- **E**ndocarditis
- **S**ick sinus syndrome

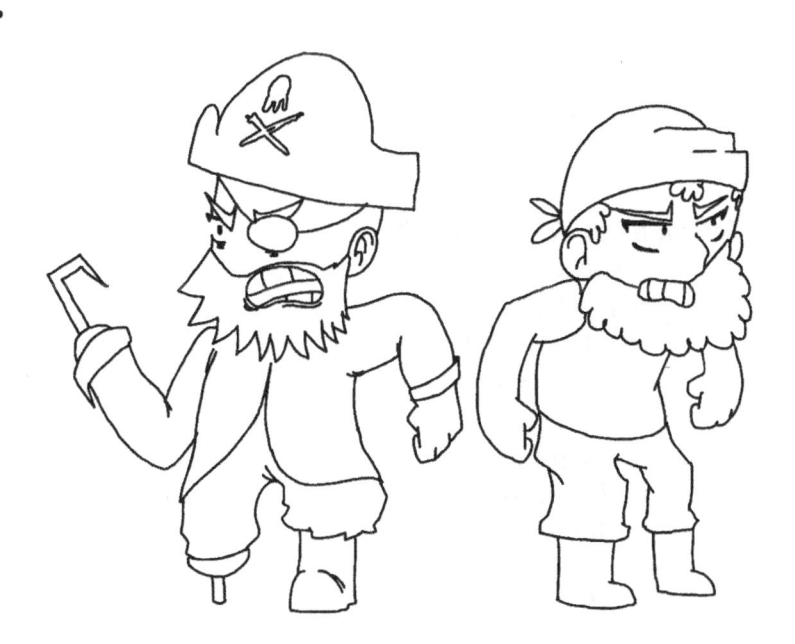

Innocent murmur features: 8 S's
- Soft
- Systolic
- Short
- Sounds (S1 and S2) normal
- Symptomless
- Special tests (normal x-ray, EKG)
- Standing/Sitting (varies with position)
- Sternal depression

Murmur attributes: IL PQRST (person has ill PQRST heart waves)
- Intensity
- Location
- Pitch
- Quality
- Radiation
- Shape
- Timing

Tetralogy of Fallot: SHOP
- Septal defect (vsd)
- Hypertrophy (right ventricular)
- Overriding aorta
- Pulmonary stenosis

Secondary causes of HTN: CHAPS
- Cushing's
- Hyperaldosteronism
- Aorta coarctation
- Pheochromocytoma
- Stenosis of renal arteries

Beta blockers 1 vs 2:
Beta 1 myocardium
Beta 2 lungs (remember 1 heart 2 lungs)

Heart sounds: All Players Earn Their Medals
- **A**ortic (Right 2nd intercostal space)
- **P**ulmonic (Left 2nd intercostal space)
- **E**rb's point (S1, S2: Left 3rd intercostal space)
- **T**ricuspid (Left lower sternal border 4th intercostal)
- **M**itral (Left 5th intercostal medial to midclavicular line)

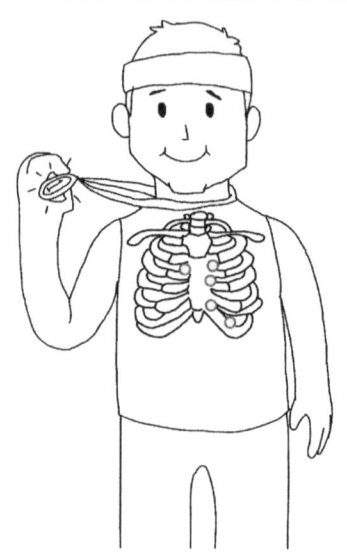

CAD risk factors: "Eating too much fatty SOFT HAM can lead to CAD
- **S**moking
- **O**besity
- **F**amily history
- **T**ype 1&2 DM
- **H**TN
- **A**ge
- **M**ale

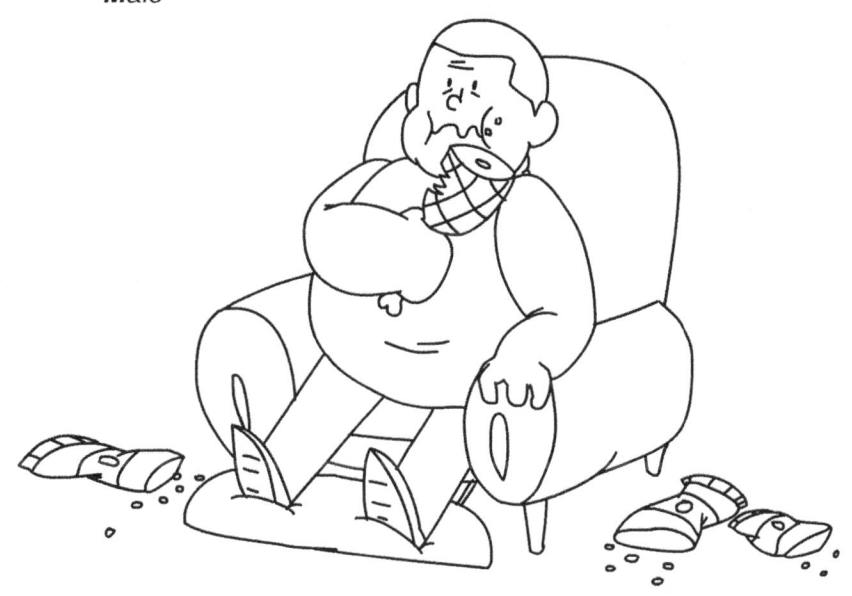

Depressed ST-segment causes: DEPRESSED ST:
- **D**rooping valve (MVP)
- **E**nlargement of LV with strain
- **P**otassium loss (hypokalemia)
- **R**eciprocal ST-depression (in Inferior wall acute myocardial infarction)
- **E**mbolism in lungs (pulmonary embolism)
- **S**ubendocardial ischemia
- **S**ubendocardial infarct
- **E**ncephalon hemorrhage (intracranial hemorrhage)
- **D**ilated cardiomyopathy
- **S**hock
- **T**oxicity (digitalis quinidine)

Chapter 7: Pulmonary

Chest x-ray interpretation: ABCDEF-
- **A**irways (hilar adenopathy or enlargement)
- **B**reast shadows/ bones (rib fractures lytic bone lesions)
- **C**ardiac silhouette (cardiac enlargement)/ Costophrenic angles (pleural effusions)
- **D**iaphragm (evidence of free air)/digestive tract
- **E**dges (apices for fibrosis pneumothorax pleural thickening or plaques)/ Extrathoracic tissues
- **F**ields (evidence of alveolar filling)/ Failure (alveolar air space disease with prominent vascularity with or without plural effusions)

ABCDEF

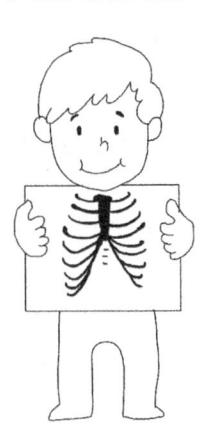

Acute stridor differential- ABCDEFGH (with fever)
- **A**bcess
- **B**acterial tracheitis
- **C**roup
- **D**iptheria
- **E**piglottis without fever:
- **F**oreign body
- **G**as (toxic gas)
- **H**ypersensitivity

Hemoptysis: causes
- **H**emmorhagic diathesis
- **E**dema
- **M**alignancy
- **O**thers [vasculitis]
- **P**ulmonary vascular abnormalities
- **T**rauma
- **Y**our treatment [anticoauglants]
- **S**tenosis (mitral)
- **I**nfection (TB, bronchitis)
- **S**cleroderma

Wheezing causes: THE ASTHMATICS
- **T**oxic fumes
- **H**ypersensitivity pneumonitis
- **E**osinophilic disease
- **A**sthma
- **S**mall airway obstruction
- **T**racheal obstruction/Large airway disease
- **H**eart failure
- **M**astocytosis/ carcinoid
- **A**naphylaxis/Allergy
- **T**hromboembolism
- **I**nfection/bronchitis
- **C**ystic fibrosis/bronchiectasis
- **S**moking/COPD

Asthma treatment: ASTHMA-
- **A**drenergic agonists
- **S**teroids
- **T**heophylline
- **H**ydration
- **M**asked oxygen
- **A**nticholinergics

Chronic Cough: "GASPS AND COUGH"
- **G**astroesophageal reflux disease
- **A**sthma
- **S**moking/chronic bronchitis
- **P**ost-infection
- **S**inusitis/post-nasal drip
- **A**ce inhibitor
- **N**eoplasm/lower airway lesion
- **D**iverticulum (esophageal)
- **C**ongestive heart failure
- **O**uter ear
- **U**pper airway obstruction
- **G**I-airway fistula
- **H**ypersensitivity/allergy

Clubbing causes: CLUBBING
- **C**yanotic heart disease
- **L**ung disease (hypox*ia, lung cancer, bronchiectasis, cystic fibrosis)*
- **U**C/Crohn's disease
- **B**iliary cirrhosis
- **B**irth defect (harmless)
- **I**nfective endocarditis
- **N**eoplasm (esp. Hodgkins)
- **G**I malabsorption

Dyspnea causes: 6 P's
- **P**ump failure
- **P**ulmonary embolus
- **P**ulmonary bronchial constriction
- **P**ossible obstruction from a foreign body
- **P**neumonia
- **P**neumothorax

Chapter 8: Gastrointestinal

Bowel anatomy: Dow Jones Industrial Average Closing Stock Report
- **D**uodenum
- **J**ejunium
- **I**leum
- **A**ppendix
- **C**olon
- **S**igmoid
- **R**ectum

Abdominal Swelling causes: 9 F's
- **F**at
- **F**eces
- **F**luid
- **F**latus
- **F**etus
- **F**ull-sized tumors
- **F**ull bladder
- **F**ibroids
- **F**alse pregnancy

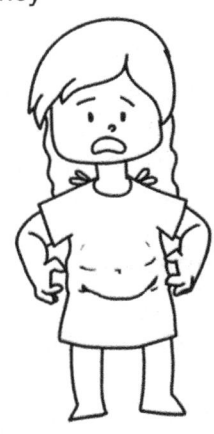

Crohn's: Crohn's has cobblestones on endoscopy

Inflammatory bowel disease (IBD): extra intestinal manifestations- A PIE SAC
- **A**phthous ulcers
- **P**yoderma gangrenosum
- **I**ritis
- **E**rythema nodosum
- **S**clerosis cholangitis
- **A**rthritis
- **C**lubbing of fingertips

Nausea & Vomiting D/Dx: A MOPING-
- **A**norexia
- **M**etabolic (DKA/Meds)
- **O**bstruction (pyloric/intestinal)
- **P**regnancy
- **I**nflammation (Pyelonephritis Cholecysto/Appendicitis/Pancreatitis, PID)
- **N**eurological (BETA)= Bleed/Encephalitis/Tumor/Abscess
- **G**astroenteritis

Gallstone risk factors: 5 f's
- **F**at
- **F**emale
- **F**air (gallstones more common in caucasians)
- **F**ertile (premenopausal- increased estrogen is thought to increase cholesterol levels in bile and decrease gallbladder contractions
- **F**orty or above

RLQ pain: APPENDICITIS
- **A**ppendicitis
- **P**elvic inflammatory disease
- **P**eriod
- **P**ancreatitis

- **E**ndometriosis
- **E**topic pregnancy
- **N**eoplasia
- **D**iverticulitis
- **I**ntussusception
- **C**yst (ovarian)
- **I**nflammatory bowel disease (Crohn's)
- **T**orsion (ovary)
- **I**rritable bowel syndrome
- **S**tones

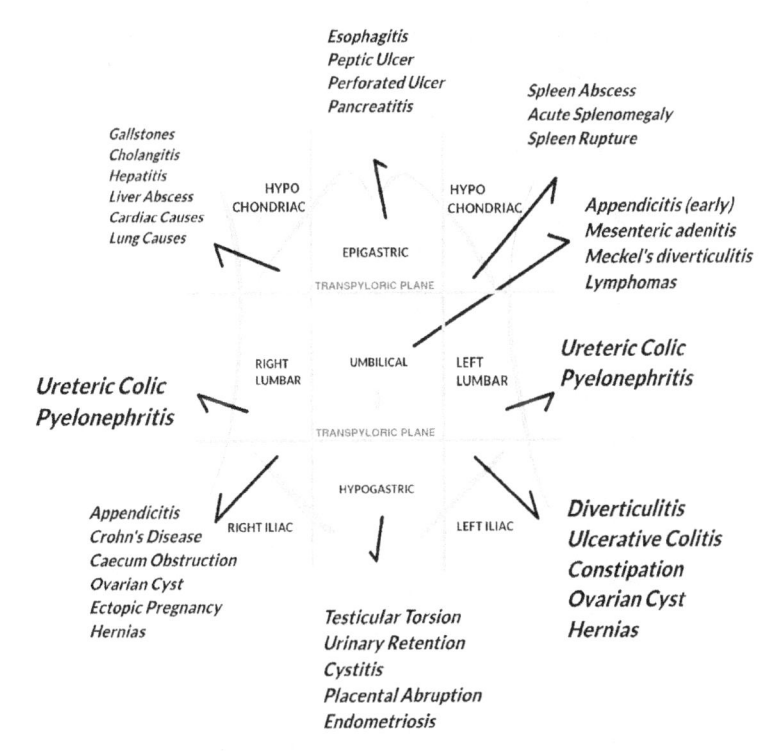

HYPOCHONDRIAC (right)
Gallstones
Cholangitis
Hepatitis
Liver Abscess
Cardiac Causes
Lung Causes

EPIGASTRIC
Esophagitis
Peptic Ulcer
Perforated Ulcer
Pancreatitis

HYPOCHONDRIAC (left)
Spleen Abscess
Acute Splenomegaly
Spleen Rupture

RIGHT LUMBAR
Ureteric Colic
Pyelonephritis

LEFT LUMBAR
Appendicitis (early)
Mesenteric adenitis
Meckel's diverticulitis
Lymphomas

Ureteric Colic
Pyelonephritis

RIGHT ILIAC
Appendicitis
Crohn's Disease
Caecum Obstruction
Ovarian Cyst
Ectopic Pregnancy
Hernias

HYPOGASTRIC
Testicular Torsion
Urinary Retention
Cystitis
Placental Abruption
Endometriosis

LEFT ILIAC
Diverticulitis
Ulcerative Colitis
Constipation
Ovarian Cyst
Hernias

TRANSPYLORIC PLANE
UMBILICAL
TRANSPYLORIC PLANE

Crohn's disease: CHRISTMAS
- **C**obblestones
- **H**igh temperature
- **R**educed lumen
- **I**ntestinal fistulae

- **S**kip lesions
- **T**ransmural (all layers, may ulcerate)
- **M**alabsorption
- **A**bdominal pain
- **S**ubmucosal fibrosis

Charcot's triad: "Charge a FEE"
- **F**ever
- **E**pigastric and RUQ pain
- **E**mesis and nausea

Vomiting differential: VOMITING
- **V**estibular disturbance/Vagal (reflex pain)
- **O**piates
- **M**igraine/Metabolic (DKA, Gastroparesis, hypercalcemia)
- **I**nfections
- **T**oxicity (cytotoxic, digitalis toxicity)
- **I**ncreased ICP, Ingested alcohol
- **N**eurogenic, psychogenic
- **G**estation

Chapter 9: Genitourinary

Causes of reversible urinary incontinence: DRIP
- **D**elirium
- **R**estricted mobility, retention
- **I**nfection, inflammation, impaction (fecal)
- **P**olyuria, pharmaceuticals

Hematuria causes: SITTT
- **S**tone
- **I**nfection
- **T**rauma
- **T**umor
- **T**uberculosis

UTI causing microorganisms: KEEPS
- **K**lebsiella
- **E**nterococcus faecalis/Enterobacter cloacae
- **E**scherichia coli
- **P**seudomonas aeroginosa/ Proteus mirabilis
- **S**taphylococcus saprophyticcus/ marcescens

Nephrotic syndrome: causes for secondary nephrotic syndrome DAVID
- *D*iabetes
- *A*myloidosis
- *V*asculitis
- *I*nfections
- *D*rugs

Prostatism symptoms: Prostate problems ain't FUN. FUN
- **F**requency
- **U**rgency
- **N**octuria

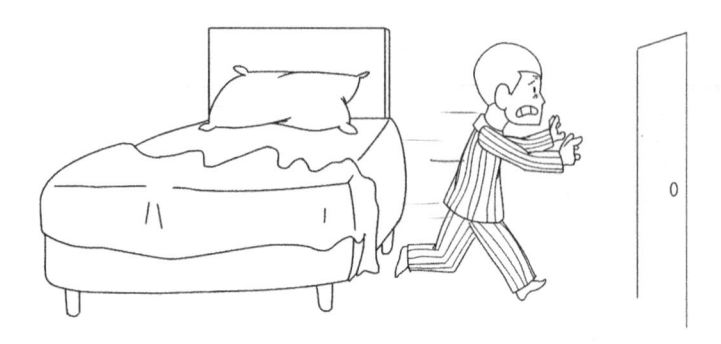

Plyelonephritis (Acute) predisposing factors: SCARRIN' UP Acute pylenephritis heals by scarrin' up the area (pyelonephritic scar)
- **S**ex (females < 40 Males > 40)
- **C**atheterization
- **A**ge (infant, elderly)
- **R**enal lesions
- **R**eflux (vescioureteral)
- **I**mmunodeficient
- **N**IDDM and IDDM
- **U**rinary obstruction
- **P**regnant

Enlarged Kidneys causes: SHAPE-
- **S**cleroderma
- **H**IV nephropathy
- **A**myloidosis
- **P**olycystic kidney disease
- **E**ndocrinopathy (diabetes)

Chapter 10: Endocrine

Cushing Syndrome: CUSHING
- **C**entral obesity/ **C**ervical fat pads, **C**ollagen fiber weakness,**C**omedones
- **U**rinary free cortisol and glucose increase
- **S**triae/Suppressed immunity
- **H**ypercortisolism/Hypertension/ Hyperglycemia/ Hirsutism
- **I**atrogenic (increased administration of corticosteroids)
- **N**onpathogenic (neoplasms)
- **G**lucose intolerance/growth retardation

Complications of diabetes: KEVINS
- **K**idney- nephropathy
- **E**ye disease- retinopathy and cataracts
- **V**ascular- coronary artery disease, cerebrovascular disease, peripheral vascular disease
- **I**nfective-TB, recurrent UTI's
- **N**euromuscular- peripheral neuropathy
- **S**kin-necrobiosis lipodica diabeticorum, granuloma annulare, diabetic dermapathy

Diabetes symptoms: 3p's of Diabetes:
- **P**olyphagia
- **P**olydipsia
- **P**olyuria

Hyperthyroid symptoms: SWEATING
- **S**weating
- **W**eight loss
- **E**motional lability
- **A**ppetite is increased
- **T**remor/Tachycardia due to A Fib
- **I**ntolerance to heat/Irregular menstruation/Irritability
- **N**ervousness
- **G**oitre and Gastrointestinal problems (loose stools/diarrhea)

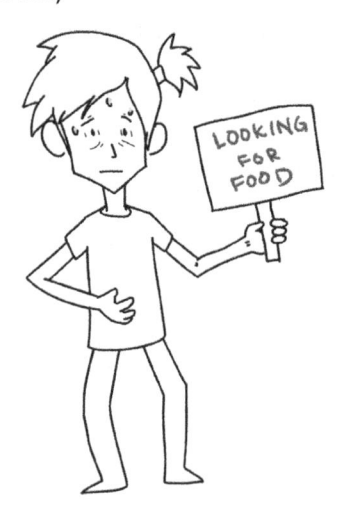

Pancreatitis causes: I GET SMASHED
- **I**diopathic
- **G**allstones
- **E**thanol
- **T**rauma
- **S**teroids
- **M**umps
- **A**utoimmune
- **S**corpion sting
- **H**yperlipdemia/hypercalcemia
- **E**RCP
- **D**rugs

Hypopituitarism: 8 I's
- **I**nvasive (primary adenoma)
- **I**nfarction (Sheehan's syndrome)
- **I**nfiltration (sarcoidosis)
- **I**atrogenic (surgery, radiation)
- **I**nfection (syphilis, TB)
- **I**njury (head trauma)
- **I**mmune (autoimmune, pregnancy)
- **I**diopathic (familial)

Causes of Addison's disease: ADDISON
- **A**utoimmune (90% of cases)
- **D**egenerative (amyloid)
- **D**rugs (ketoconazole)
- **I**nfections (TB, HIV)
- **S**econdary (low ACTH); hypopituitarism
- **O**thers (adrenal bleeding)
- **N**eoplasia (secondary carcinoma)

Symptoms of hypothyroidism: "MOM'S SO TIRED"
- **M**emory loss
- **O**besity
- **M**alar flush/Menorrhagia
- **S**lowness
- **S**kin and hair become dry
- **O**nset is gradual
- **T**ired
- **I**ntolerance to cold
- **R**aised blood pressure
- **E**nergy levels are low
- **D**epressed

Hypothyroidism is 10 times more common in females and occurs mainly in middle life.

Chapter 11: Hematology

Anemia causes: ANEMIA
- **A**nemia of chronic diseases
- **N**o folate or B12
- **E**thanol
- **M**arrow failure and hemoglobinopathies
- **I**ron deficient
- **A**cute and chronic blood loss

Causes of splenomegaly: CHINA
- **C**ongestive
- **H**ematological
- **I**nfectious
- **N**eoplastic
- **A**utoimmune

Chronic liver disease: ABCDEFGHIJ
- **A**sterixis (liver flap)/ascites/ankle edema/atrophy of testicles
- **B**ruising/BP
- **C**lubbing/color change of nails; white (leuconychia)
- **D**upuytren's contracture
- **E**rythema (palmar)/encephalopathy
- **F**etor hepaticus
- **G**ynocomastia
- **H**epato-splenomegaly
- **I**ncreased size of parotid
- **J**aundice

Spleen Dimensions: 1,3,5,7,9,11:
The spleen is **1** inch x **3** inches x **5** inches. Weight is **7** ounces. It lies underneath ribs **9** through **11**

Microcytic anemia causes: ABCDEF
- **A**lcohol + liver disease
- **B**12 deficiency
- **C**ompensatory reticulocytosis (blood loss and hemolysis)
- **D**rug (cytotoxic and AZT)/Dysplasia (marrow problems)
- **E**ndocrine (hypothyroidism)
- **F**olate Deficiency/Fetus (pregnancy)

Raynaud's disease causes: BAD CT
- **B**lood disorders (polycythemia)
- **A**rterial (atherosclerosis
- **B**uerger's)
- **D**rugs (eg. Beta Blockers)
- **C**onnective tissue disorders (rheumatoid arthritis, SLE)
- **T**raumatic (eg. vibratory injury)

Splenomegaly causes: CHICAGO
- **C**ancer
- **H**em onc (blood cancers)
- **I**nfection
- **C**ongestion (portal HTN)
- **A**utoimmune (RA, SLE)
- **G**lycogen storage disorders
- **O**thers (amyloidosis)

Folate deficiency causes: A FOLIC DROP
- **A**lcoholism
- **F**olic Acid antagonists
- **O**ral contraceptives
- **L**ow dietary intake
- **I**nfection with Giardia
- **C**eliac sprue
- **D**ilantin
- **R**elative folate deficiency
- **O**ld

- **P**regnant

Sickle cell disease Signs: SICKLE
- **S**plenomegaly/Sludging
- **I**nfection
- **C**holelithiasis
- **K**idney – hematuria
- **L**iver congestion/Leg ulcers
- **E**ye changes

Symptoms and signs: LEUKEMIA
- **L**ight skin (pallor)
- **E**nergy decreased/Enlarged spleen, liver, lymph nodes
- **U**nderweight
- **K**idney failure
- **E**xcess heat (fever)
- **M**ottled skin (hemorrhage)
- **I**nfections
- **A**nemia

Chapter 12: Immunology

DeGeorge Syndrome (features): The disease of T's
- **T**hird and 4th pharyngeal pouch absent
- **T**wenty-Two chromosome
- **T**-cells absent
- **T**etany: hypocalcemia

Celiac Sprue features: CELIAC
- **C**ell-mediated autoimmune disease
- **E**uropean descent
- **L**ymphocytes in Lamina propria/ Lymphoma risk
- **I**ntolerance of gluten (wheat)
- **A**trophy of villi in small intestine/Abnormal D-xylose test
- **C**hildhood presentation

Sjogren Syndrome: morphology "Jog through the MAPLES":
- **M**outh dry
- **A**rthritis
- **P**arotids enlarged
- **L**ymphoma
- **E**yes dry
- **S**icca (primary) or secondary.

Acromegaly symptoms: ABCDEF
- **A**rthralgia/Arthritis
- **B**lood pressure raised
- **C**arpal tunnel syndrome
- **D**iabetes
- **E**nlarged organs

- Field (visual) defect

Gynecomastia causes: GYNECOMASTIA
- **G**enetic Gender disorder (Klinefelter)
- **Y**oung boy (pubertal)
- **N**eonate*
- **E**strogen
- **C**irrhosis/Cimetidine/Ca Channel blockers
- **O**ld age
- **M**arijuana
- **A**lcoholism
- **S**pironolactone
- **T**umors (testicular and adrenal)
- **I**soniazid/Inhibition of testosterone
- **A**ntineoplastic (Alkylating Agents)/Antifungals (keto-conazole) *indicates physiologic cause

Goodpasture's Syndrome: GoodPasture has
- **G**lomerulonephritis
- **P**nuemonitits

SLE factors that make it active: UV PRISM
- **UV** (sunshine)
- **P**regnancy
- **R**educed drug (e.g. steroid)
- **I**nfection
- **S**tress
- **M**edication

Gout: GOUT
- **G**ents
- **O**verweight
- **U**ric acid elevated
- **T**ophi- pathognomonic sign

Hypersensitivity type IV example:
"Poison **IV**y causes type **IV** hypersensitivity."

Lupus Signs and Symptoms: SOAP BRAIN
- **S**erositis [pleuritis, pericarditis]
- **O**ral ulcers
- **A**rthritis
- **P**hotosensitivity
- **B**lood [all are low- anemia, leukopenia, thrombocytopenia]
- **R**enal [protein]
- **A**NA
- **I**mmunologic [DS DNA, etc.]
- **N**eurologic [psych, seizures]

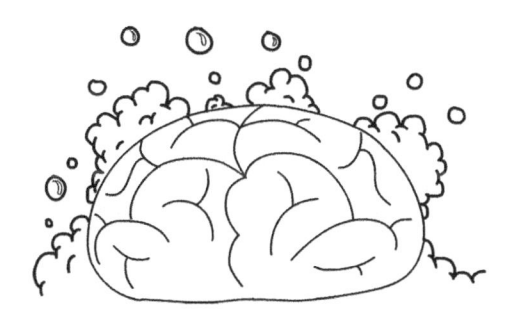

Polycythemia Vera: PRV
- **P**lethora/Pruritis
- **R**inging in ears
- **V**isual blurriness

Hypersensitivity reaction ACID
- **Type 1** - **Allergic,** IgE mediated; quick onset after exposure **Allergic** (bee stings, latex, certain medications)
- **Type II** - **Cytotoxic**/antibody-mediated Cytotoxic (Hemolytic reactions, Goodpasture syndrome, Hyperacute graft rejection)
- **Type III** - **Immune** complex/IgG/IgM mediated Immune complex deposition (hypersensitive pneumonitis, systemic lupus erythematosus, polyarteritis nodosa, serum sickness)
- **Type IV** - **Delayed** or cell-mediated Delayed (chronic graft rejections, PPD test, latex, nickel, poisonous ivy)

Chapter 13: Musculoskeletal

Carpal bones: "So long to Pinky - Here Comes The Thumb."
- Scaphoid
- Lunate
- Triqutrum
- Pisforme
- Hamate
- Capitate
- Trapezoid
- Trapezium

Sprains and strains treatment: RICE
- Rest
- Ice
- Compression
- Elevation

Carpal Tunnel syndrome causes: MEDIAN TRAP
- Myxoedema
- Edema (heart failure, OCP, Pre-menstrual)
- Diabetes mellitus
- Idiopathic
- Acromegaly
- Neoplasia
- Trauma
- Rheumatoid arthritis
- Amyloidosis
- Pregnancy

Fractures: GO C3PO
- **G**reenstick
- **O**pen
- **C**omplete
- **C**losed
- **C**omminuted
- **P**artial
- **O**ther

Fall potential causes- Illness: I'VE FALLEN
- **I**llness
- **V**estibular
- **E**nvironmental
- **F**eet/Footwear
- **A**lcohol and drugs
- **L**ow BP
- **L**ow 02 sats
- **E**ars/Eyes
- **N**europathy

Short stature causes: RETARD HEIGHT
- **R**ickets
- **E**ndocrine (cretinism, hypopituitarism, Cushing's)
- **T**urner syndrome
- **A**chrondroplasia
- **R**espiratory (suppurative lung disease)
- **D**own syndrome
- **H**ereditary
- **E**nvironmental (post irradiation, post infection)
- **I**UGR
- **G**I (malabsorption)
- **H**eart (congenital heart disease)
- **T**wisted backbone (scoliosis)

Back pain D/D: LIMCOTS
- **L**umbar spinal stenosis
- **I**ntervertebral disc herniation
- **M**ultiple Myeloma/ Mets (Prostate, Breast, Lung)
- **C**auda equina syndrome/ Cancer
- **O**steoporosis/Osteoarthritis
- **T**rauma/TB
- **S**train/Sprain

Arm Fracture Differences
- Colle's vs Smith's fracture: Colle's fracture: arm in fall position makes a "C" shape

Smith's fracture: arm in fall position makes a "S" shape

Chapter 14: Reproductive

Oral contraceptives side effects: CONTRACEPTIVES
- **C**holestatic jaundice
- **O**edema (corneal)
- **N**asal congestion
- **T**hyroid dysfunction
- **R**aised BP
- **A**cne/ Alopecia/Anemia
- **C**erebrovascular disease
- **E**levated blood sugar
- **P**orphyria/Pigmentation/ Pancreatitis
- **T**hromboembolism
- **I**ntracranial hypertension
- **V**omiting (progesterone only)
- **E**rythema nodosum/Extrapyramidal effects
- **S**ensitivity to light

Preeclampsia classic triad: PREeclampsia
- **P**roteinuria
- **R**ising blood pressure
- **E**dema

Menopause – long-term effects: CONU
- **C**ardiovascular disease: IHD stroke, arterial disease
- **O**steoporosis: accelerated bone loss leading to osteoporosis and pathological, fractures
- **N**eurological: Alzheimer's disease
- **U**rogenital atrophy: loss of pelvic floor muscle tone

Premenopausal symptoms: HAVOC
- **H**ot flashes
- **A**trophy of vagina
- **V**aginal dryness
- **O**steoporosis
- **C**AD

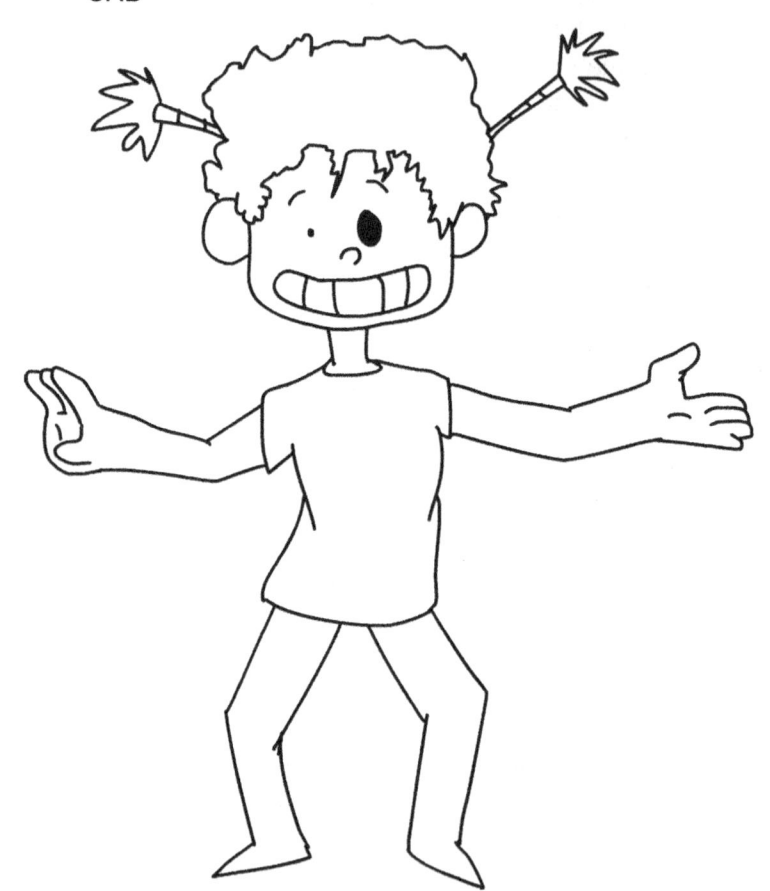

Dysfunctional uterine bleeding (DUB): 3 major causes
- **D**on't ovulate (anovulation 90% of causes)
- **U**nusual corpus luteum activity (prolonged or insufficient)

- **B**irth control pills (since increases progesterone-estrogen ratio)

Placenta-crossing Substances: WANT My Hot Dog
- **W**astes
- **A**ntibodies
- **N**utrients
- **T**eratogens
- **M**icroorganisms
- **H**ormones, HIV
- **D**rugs

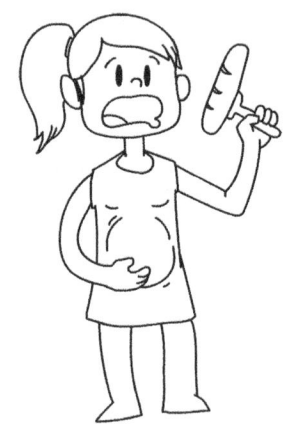

BCP warnings: ACHES
- **A**bdominal pain
- **C**hest pain
- **H**eadache
- **E**ye (blurry vision)
- **S**harp leg pain

IUD side-effects: PAINS
- **P**eriod that is late
- **A**bdominal cramps
- **I**ncrease in body temperature
- **N**oticeable vaginal discharge
- **S**potting

Impotence causes: PLANE
- **P**sychogenic: performance anxiety
- **L**ibido: decreased with androgen deficiency, drugs
- **A**utonomic neuropathy: impede blood flow redirection
- **N**itric oxide deficiency: impaired synthesis, decreased blood pressure
- **E**rectile reserve: can't maintain an erection

Male erectile dysfunction biologic causes: MED
- **M**edicines (propranalol, methyldopa, SSRI)
- **E**thanol
- **D**iabetes mellitus

Teratogens: Placenta-crossing organisms: TORCHES
- **T**oxoplasma
- **O**thers (parvovirus, listeria)
- **R**ubella
- **C**MV
- **H**erpes simplex
    - **H**erpes zoster (varicella)
    - **H**epatitis B,C,E
- **E**nteroviruses
- **S**yphilis

Abdominal pain during pregnancy causes: LARA CROFT
- **L**abor
- **A**bruption of placenta
- **R**upture (e.g. Ectopic/uterus)
- **A**bortion
- **C**holestasis
- **R**ectus sheath hematoma
- **O**varian tumor
- **F**ibroids
- **T**orsion of uterus

Trichomaniasis features: 5F's
- **F**lagella
- **F**rothy discharge
- **F**ishy odor (sometimes)
- **F**ornication
- **F**lagyl (Metronidazole) Rx

Menopause – symptoms: FSH > 20 IU/L
Remember that this is the most accurate blood test for confirmation of menopause!
- **F**lushes (hot) /**F**emale genitalia (vaginal) dryness and burning
- **S**weats at night
- **H**eadaches
- **I**nsomnia
- **U**rge incontinence
- **L**ibido decreases

Infertility – causes and risk factors, INFERTILE (in females)
- **I**diopathic
- **N**o ovulation – PCOS, menopause, pituitary disease, thyroid disorders
- **F**ibroids – physical hindrance
- **E**ndometriosis
- **R**egular bleeding pattern disrupted – oligo/amenorrhoea
- **T**ubal disease leading to blocked/damaged cilia
- **I**ncreasing age >35 years
- **L**arge size – obesity
- **E**xcessive weight loss – anorexia nervosa

Chapter 15: Pediatrics

Croup symptoms: 3 S's
- **S**tridor
- **S**ubglottic swelling
- **S**eal (barking cough)

Presentation of impetigo: IMPETIGO
- **I**nfection w/staph aureus, strep pyrogens, or both. Mostly in young children
- **P**articularly around nose and surrounding parts of the face
- **E**rythematous base with honey-colored crusts
- **T**reat with topical antibiotics such as fusidic acid or bacitracinfor honey-colored lesions
- **I**ndividuals are highly contagious from skin-to-skin contact; improve hygiene; do not share towels
- **G**ram stain and culture of swab diagnostic
- **O**ral flucloxacillin required for widespread impetigo

Signs of Kawasaki's: CLEAR
- **C**onjunctivitis
- **L**ymphadenopathy lips
- **E**xtremity changes (peeling or bright red palms and soles)
- **A**neurysms
- **R**ash

Puberty events: "The Prime Minister"
- **Th**elarche
- **P**ubarche
- **M**enarche

Rash time of onset after fever: "Really Sick Children Must Take No Exercise."
- Day 1: Rubella
- Day 2: Scarlet fever/ Smallpox
- Day 3: Chickenpox
- Day 4: Measles (will see Koplik spots one day prior to rash)
- Day 5: Typhus & rickettsia (variable)
- Day 6: Nothing
- Day 7: Enteric fever (samonella)

Breastfeeding – advantages: PACES
- **P**sychological satisfaction
- **A**nti-infective property/Atopic disorders (decreases risk)
- **C**onvenient
- **E**xpenseless, i.e. free
- **S**timulates growth and development

Breastfeeding – disadvantages: KIDS
- **K** and D vitamin deficiency
- **I**nfection transmission risk eg: HIV
- **D**rugs excreted in milk
- **S**tressful and tiring for mother

Lead poisoning: presentation – ABCDEFG
- **A**nemia
- **B**asophilic stripping
- **C**olicky pain
- **D**iarrhea
- **E**ncephalopathy
- **F**oot drop
- **G**ums (lead line)

Chapter 16: Psychosocial

Depression (major episode characteristics) SPACE DIGS:
- **S**leep disruption
- **P**sychomotor retardation
- **A**ppetite change
- **C**oncentration loss
- **E**nergy loss
- **D**epressed mood
- **I**nterest wanes
- **G**uilt
- **S**uicidal tendencies.

States of dying: "Death Always Brings Great Acceptance"
- **D**enial
- **A**nger
- **B**argaining
- **G**rieving
- **A**cceptance

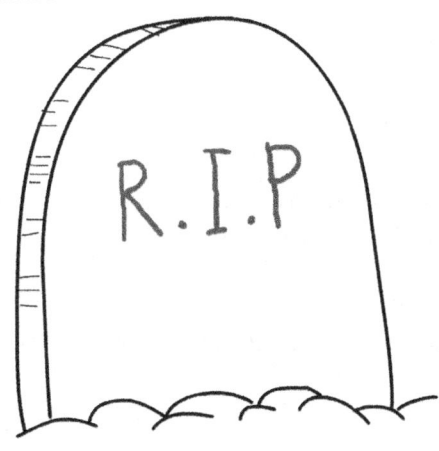

Fatigue: MAD HIP
- **M**alignancy
- **A**buse
- **D**epression
- **H**yperthyroidism
- **I**nfection
- **P**TSD

Suicide risk factors: SAD PERSONS
- **S**ex: male
- **A**ge: young, elderly
- **D**epression
- **P**revious suicide attempts
- **E**thanol and other drugs
- **R**eality testing/ Rational though (loss of)
- **S**ocial support lacking
- **O**rganized suicide plan
- **N**o spouse
- **S**ickness/Stated future intent

Lethargy causes: FATIGUED:
- **F**at/Food (poor diet)
- **A**nemia
- **T**umor
- **I**nfection (HIV, endocarditis)
- **G**eneral joint or liver disease
- **U**remia
- **E**ndocrine (Addison's, myxedema)
- **D**iabetes/Depression/Drugs

CAGE questionnaire:
- Have you ever felt you should? **C**ut down on your drinking?
- Have people **A**NNOYED you by criticizing your drinking?
- Have you ever felt bad or **G**UILTY about your drinking?

- Have you ever had a drink first thing in the morning to steady your nerves or get rid of a hangover (**EYE-OPENER**)?

Chapter 17: Pharmacology

Beta 1 selective blockers "BEAM me up, Scotty":
- **B**eta 1 blockers:
- **E**smolol
- **A**tenolol
- **M**etoprolol

B vitamin names: "The Rhythm Nearly Proved Contagious"
- **T**hiamine (B1)
- **R**iboflavin (B2)
- **N**iacin (B3)
- **P**yridoxine (B6)
- **C**obalamin (B12)

Fat Soluble vitamins: KADE
- **K** Vitamin
- **A** Vitamin
- **D** Vitamin
- **E** Vitamin

NSAID contraindications
- **N**ursing and pregnancy
- **S**erious bleeding
- **A**llergy/Asthma/Angioedema
- **I**mpaired renal function
- **D**rug (anticoagulant)

Serotonin syndrome components: Causes **HARM**:
- **H**yperthermia
- **A**utonomic instability (delirium)
- **R**igidity
- **M**yoclonus

MAOIs: indications MAOI'S: Listed in decreasing order of importance. Note MAOI is inside **MelAnchOlIc**.
- **M**elancholic [classic name for atypical depression]
- **A**nxiety
- **O**besity disorders [anorexia, bulimia]
- **I**magined illnesses [hypochondria]
- **S**ocial phobias

K+ increasing agents K-BANK:
- **K**-sparing diuretic
- **B**eta blocker
- **A**CE Inhibitor
- **N**SAID
- **K** supplement

Antibiotics contraindicated during pregnancy MCAT:
- **M**etronidazole
- **C**hloramphenicol
- **A**minoglycoside
- **T**etracycline

Steroid side effects CUSHINGOID:
- **C**ataracts
- **U**lcers
- **S**kin: striae, thinning, bruising
- **H**ypertension/ Hirsutisim/ Hyperglycemia
- **I**nfections
- **N**ecrosis (avascular necrosis of the femoral head)
- **G**lycosuria
- **O**steoporosis, obesity
- **I**mmunosuppression
- **D**iabetes

Alternate:
Steroids- side effects: BECLOMETHASONE:
- **B**uffalo hump
- **E**asy bruising
- **C**ataracts
- **L**arger appetite
- **O**besity
- **M**oonface
- **E**uphoria
- **T**hin arms & legs
- **H**ypertension/ **H**yperglycemia
- **A**vascular necrosis of femoral head
- **S**kin thinning
- **O**steoporosis
- **N**egative nitrogen balance
- **E**motional liability

Chapter 18: Top 25 Drugs in Family Practice

1. Synthroid
2. Crestor
3. Nexium
4. Ventolin HFA
5. Advair Diskus
6. Cymbalta
7. Diovan
8. Vyvanse
9. Lantus Solostar
10. Lyrica
11. Spiriva Handihaler
12. Lantus
13. Celebrex
14. Januvia
15. Abilify
16. Namenda
17. Viagra
18. Zetia
19. Cialis
20. Nasonex
21. Suboxone
22. Bystolic
23. Symbicort
24. Flovent HFA
25. Oxycontin

Sources

www.answers.medchrome.com
www.asha.org
www.dermmnemonics.org
www.doctorshangout.com/page/pharmacology-mnemonics
www.medical-institution.com
www.medscape.com/viewarticle/825053#vp_2
www.nursebuff.com
www.prep4usmle.com
www.quizlet.com
www.scribd.com
www.slideshare.net/sarosem1/anatomy-mnemonics-guide
www.studynow.com
www.wikepedia.com

About the Author

Nachole Johnson is a nurse practitioner who loves educating and inspiring other nurses to succeed in life. She has authored numerous blogs and articles for Minority Nurse Magazine and dailynurse.com. She is the author of multiple books including *You're a Nurse and Want to Start Your Own Business? The Complete Guide,* published under ReNursing Publishing Company. She is also founder of ReNursing Career Consulting, a company dedicated to empowering nurses. Learn more at amazon.com/author/nacholejohnson.

Other Books By Nachole Johnson

Nurse Practitioner School and Beyond: http://amzn.to/2d8viiN

Business Ideas for the Entrepreneurial Nurse: http://amzn.to/2d3HG8H

You're a Nurse and Want to Start Your Own Business: http://amzn.to/1knq4Sj

The Financially Savvy Nurse Practitioner: http://amzn.to/2jZvpoy

Made in the USA
Columbia, SC
19 January 2024